Sex Positions

100 Sex Positions to Try before You Die: The Ultimate Sex Guide for His & Her Pleasure

Table of Contents

Introduction

Congratulations on downloading *Sex Positions: 100 Sex Positions to Try before You Die – The Ultimate Guide for His & Her Pleasure* and thank you so much for doing so! You are on the fast track to learning new and improved ways to enhance your sexual game with your partner.

The following chapters in this book will hit every major topic when it comes to having the ultimately BEST sex of your life, whether it is with your spouse, significant other or a one-night stand. The chapters in this book cover:

- Techniques for foreplay to get each of your riled up and ready to get down and dirty
- Approaches for trying brand new sex positions
- Mastering the location of her G-Spot and how to pleasure it
- Ways to last longer while in the sack
- How to please your man in bed
- How to please your woman in bed
- Techniques and new tricks to have the best oral sex
- How to give heightening sexual massages
- And much more!

Why live your life having mediocre sex when you have the ability to unlock so many different sexual secrets with the power of this one book? What are you waiting for?! Get to reading so you can be on your way to pleasuring the love of your life, or impressing the individuals you take home from plethora of parties!

There are plenty of books on sex and how to sexually please your partner on the market, so thanks again for choosing this one! Every effort was made to ensure it is full of as much useful information as possible, please enjoy!

Foreplay Techniques

As human beings, we build romantic foundations on the core aspect of being able to physically bond with the one we have deep connections with. Besides the feel good sensations we get from taking the time to stimulate and arouse our partner for sexual intercourse, the process of foreplay also increases emotional connectedness with our spouse. No matter what you plan on doing in bed at the time, foreplay is a powerful part of making any sexual experience more pleasurable.

Importance of Foreplay

There are some that see this part as more of a chore than an experience all on its own, especially men towards women. It is no secret that the opposite sexes do not always see eye to eye when it comes to sexual prelude. Get that idea out of your mind right now! Fondling before intercourse is more than just a tried and true way to get him erect and get her slippery wet. View it more as the delicious, intricate act of lovemaking before you move on to make the genitals feel good.

Just the mere thought of sex alone can arouse men to the point of erection, but women are usually not so lucky. Foreplay serves a vital purpose in the bedroom, and should be taken pretty seriously. It has both emotional and physical purposes, as it prepares the minds and bodies for intercourse. In fact, foreplay has direct ties to the longevity of sex as well. As you do physical things with one another to build up to sex, the act of sex is WAY better, and leads to exceptional orgasm from both sexes. Foreplay also provides the energy to maintain intercourse for longer periods of time, which is obviously a plus on both ends!

Foreplay is important when having sex in any type of relationship, whether it's a friends with benefits type of deal, or a long-term relationship. It is even more crucial for married couples who have the loads of stress from work, kids, finances and other life struggles. Foreplay assists in maintaining an intimate connection with your spouse, which flows into many aspects of the relationship as a whole. Couples must remember that foreplay is a TEAM effort, not just the responsibility of one partner or the other.

Foreplay Do's & Don'ts

It is great to be sexually creative with your partner, but there are some relatively key things you need to keep in mind, for despite your best efforts, it can be easy to turn your spouse off when you are trying your best to turn them on in the heat of the moment.

The DO'S of Foreplay

Know their hotspots – Do not just set your main focus on the penis or vagina. Every individual has a different set of hotspots that will get them really riled up if touched correctly. You can lick, nibble, kiss, stroke and caress these areas in any way you see fit, as long as the person you are doing it to enjoys it. You are essentially turning the "on" switch to the green light.

It is also important to know where hotspots are, especially as a starting point. This is vital when you are just getting to know your partner sexually. Here are some hints!

- **Lips** – Knowing the proper ways to kiss one another is an experience all in itself. The border surrounding the lips is extremely sensitive. Lightly tracing your fingertip around the edges of their mouth will make them feel a ticklish, tingly type feeling. When you are kissing, use the tip of your tongue to playfully trace the edge of their mouth.
- **Indention between neck and collar bone** – The skin is thinner in this area, so any sort of sensation will be much stronger. The movement of your mouth, for example, over this sensitive area will send heat from your breath, as well as relaxation, resulting in getting turned on.
- **Sides of torso** – The area from the bottom of the rib cage all the way to the hips is filled with powerful nerves

3

that connect directly to the clitoris and the penis. So, when stimulated, those muscles kick into gear and contract. Firmer touches will get you farther here, since this area is more ticklish than others.

- **Base of the spine** – There is a nifty little knob-like rift at the base of the spine that is full of major nerves that withhold plenty of pleasure potential. If you start within the shoulder blades, and work your hands down in a kneading type of motion, once you get to the lower back lightly spiral your fingertips over the base with a soft touch. That will get them going for sure!
- **Thighs** – Any sexual person KNOWS that the thighs are where many explosive nerves are located, especially towards the top of the inner thigh. Playing with different touches here will quickly do the trick of turning them on.
- **Other areas of arousal**:
  - Nipples
  - Neck
  - Ears
  - Back
  - Buttocks
  - Feet
  - Armpits

Be innovative while you are on the mission in exploring your partner's body. Everyone is different, and likes to have certain erogenous areas touched variously. Do not just rely on well known hotspots either. Take your spouse by surprise and venture into unexpected places, for that in itself is a great turn on!

Mix it up – Doing the same routine over and over becomes awfully boring very quickly. That is why it's vital to ingenious in the ways you conduct foreplay. Even if you are a tad bit shy in trying something different, your partner will pay you back ten fold and appreciate your efforts.

Try:

- Teasing your sexual partner with your lips, your mouth, by touch or with creative sex props, such as textured gloves or feathers
- Use a new kind of lube for an entirely new sensation

The key here is to spice things up so sex does not become predictable. The element of surprise is a turn on all on its own.

Spoil one another – Nothing feels nicer than being spoiled by your spouse. And it is vital to take the time and energy to do so for one another. Take ample time to kiss, cuddle and stroke each other without demanding anything further. Get out the massage oil and give your partner a relaxing and much needed massage. Sensual touching feels amazing and can be an easy way to get your partner in the mood for sex.

The DON'TS of Foreplay

Rush – Foreplay is an important part of any kind of sexual play, especially for females, for they need more time to really get into the mood, and for their vaginas to get properly lubricated for the men's already erect penis. Otherwise, sex will not be as pleasurable and can potentially be painful. So if you are looking for a cringe-free sex session, dedicate time to it.

Overdo it – Foreplay is amazing and a crucial part that leads up to mind blowing sex. Slow and passionate buildup is super hot, but only to a point. If you continue to drag foreplay out, men could potentially ejaculate before he ever even gets inside you! No, there is no "set" amount of time for foreplay, because everyone is uniquely different. There will also be some days that you want to participate in foreplay more than others.

Happens only in bed – Foreplay and sex in general does not always have to be conducted in a horizontal fashion. It can also start much earlier during the course of the day, perhaps when you catch one another's eyes and stare into them deeply, or accidental touches, or surprise passionate kisses. Flirting and teasing one another while not in the midst of a bedroom counts as foreplay too! Just the mere fact of letting someone know that you are attracted to them and want to make love to them later on is a HUGE turn on.

The Most Important Part of Foreplay

The most important piece of foreplay cannot be categorized, for it is one of the most crucial parts of any relationship, and that is communication. Whether it be physical, mental or verbal. During the course of both foreplay and sex, pay attention to your spouse's body language. If they do not seem to like whatever you are doing to them, stop. If they communicate something they are embarrassed to tell you, listen with intent and no judgment. Neither one of you are psychics, so you must tell one another how you feel. This also proves true during actual foreplay and intercourse time. If you do not like the way something feels, speak up! If your partner is just barely missing a spot that they are touching, tell them. You will both enjoy the time spent together sexually more if you learn to communicate your desires on a regular basis.

Also, HAVE FUN! Foreplay is a time to be creative and to get your partner and yourself in the mood for the swing of things later on! Communication creates a comfortable bond with your sexual partners, and feeling non-judged and comfortable with the person you are so close to helps in pushing that ON button!

Powerful Foreplay Techniques

Take control – Most often, men play the dominant role when it comes to activities within the bedroom. But occassionally, it is beyond sexy for the women to grab the dominance by the horns and run with it! Some ways to take authority in the sack are:

- Demanding them to do things like stripping off his clothing or going down on you
- Straddling him with his hands tied behind his head
- Taking over how you both move around during intercourse. Command what positions you want to sex them in.

Kiss more than the mouth – Lips are an obvious place to place yours upon. To truly spice things up, you must take your mouth on adventures up and down the body, places where you lips have never touched before.
Other places to kiss:

- If pants are off, kiss your partner above the knee and work your way to their crotch
- If their top is absent, kiss them from their neck all the way down to their genital area. You can do this quickly or slowly, whichever you prefer. The slower you perform this motion, the more anticipation builds up. You can then give them oral at this point.
- Kiss lightly around their ears, neck and cheeks, for these areas are very sensitive to the touch.

Grope and caress – Especially during times when sex has not been able to occur because of busy schedules and such, when you finally get the chance to be phyical, the tension that has built up over time makes you both eager to rip one another's clothing off. Despite how great that is and the boiling anticipation that you both have residing inside of you, making the time to take things slow will make the inital sex a LOT of fun. Groping, rubbing and caressing on the outside of each other's clothing makes desperation much more exciting.
Here are some movements you can make:

- While kissing them, put your arm under theirs so you have the power to grab and pull them up closer to you
- Straddle them while fooling around, rub their crotches to tease them
- If you are standing, pinch, caress or rub their buttocks
- Take a hand and slowly run it along the inside of one of their legs, just above the knee. When you get to their crotch area, massage there softly and slowly

Build up tension – Building tension between the two of you is actual not considered a physical aspect of foreplay, it is a mental one. Sex is both a mental and physical encounter. Here are some ways to successfully build the right amounts of tension that will lead you to mind blowing intercourse:

- Brush your hand over their sensitve areas like their crotch and buttocks.
- Use teasing commentary such as *"If I was alone with you right now I would pounce on you!"*
- Send them naughty texts such as *"I can't wait to get my mouth around you this evening ;)"*

Ask what turns them on – Do not be shy, go ahead and ask what your spouse likes during sex, as well as what really turns them on. In fact, most females really appreciate this, for it means that the man has taken the opportunity to really tune into her sexual needs and desires. If she notices that you are taking the extra time to really please her, she is more likely to return the favor to you ten fold later!

Now that we got foreplay out of the way, now it is time to turn to the next chapter and explore some exciting new sexual positions!

Arousing Sex Positions

There are not many individuals among the human race who do not like or appreciate sex. I am sure there are some that would gladly take a week off of work and push aside responsibilities for sex if they could, trust me. Sex is kind of like a feel good drug that has a lot more great side effects than any of those nasty drugs out there, so why NOT do it more often?

Sex is about variety, and having an assortment of different sexual positions that you know how to conduct under your belt is a good asset to have. There are literally hundreds of contrasting sexual positions out there that we can either choose to ignore, or that we can choose to embrace to possibly have the most incredibly amazing sex we have ever felt! It does not matter if you are greatly experienced in the world of intercourse, or are a newbie to what it can be all about. To jump start your creativity in mastering your sexual imagination, this chapter is filled with some of the best sex position to improve your sex life!

Missionary Positions

Missionary is the most traditional ways to intervene in intercourse, for it is the most personable of the positions. There are a few variations to spice up this vanilla-type position.

Coital Alignment Technique – Also known as the 'Perfect Position" the CAT is all about the proper elevation to seek the right position. To perform this, you and your partner need to start out in the regular missionary position, then flatten your torso as your partner arches their legs and rests them around your butt. You are then hitting the clitoris with the perfect amount of pressure to assist in making her orgasm quicker. You will need to be thrusting gently deeply in and out to ensure maximum pleasure for both of you.

Pancake – Start with your torso in a vertical position and have your spouse put their legs on your shoulders. Descend until you have essentially folded your partner in half. This position is highly intimate, while also allowing you to have most of the thrusting power. Ensure that your partner is flexible enough to be able to perform this position; otherwise it can be rather painful and unpleasant.

Spread Eagle – This position is perhaps the most intimate, and it requires you to get in touch with your kinkier side with some bondage. Lay your partner on their back and make them spread their legs apart. Tie their wrists to their ankles. You then have them in a place where you are in total control.

Viennese Oyster – This one requires a bit of flexibility, but one partner places both their ankles up to their head, exposing their genitals as their body is folded up into the shape of an oyster. This can be used for extremely deep penetration.

Doggy-Style Positions

Doggy-style positions involve one of the partners having a lot of control over the other, usually the men versus the women. They are less intimate, but allow for all rots of possibilities, as each person involved can be lying down, kneeling or standing. These positions also allow both partners to be able to stimulate the clitoris, so there is not much not to like!

The Original – The classic doggy-style positioning is a treat for millions of couples, and is the main female submissive position that lets the man be in total control. In this form, you allow your partner to position themselves on all fours on a bed or other surface. You kneel behind them, enter them from behind and hold onto their hips. The pace at which you penetrate them is up to the both of you. Doggy-style allows plenty of room for the dominator to be kinky, and can be rough such as hair pulling or spanking.

Bedside Doggy – This one defies the odds of the classic doggy-style by placing the female or non-dominate party stand and bend, as the man or dominate party kneels on the bed or platform. Have your partner back up to you, and bend them over about 90 degrees. Then thrust away.

Back Door Plank – This position is as the G-Spot and A-Spot access or, but is it highly comfortable for the female or non-dominant party. Let your partner lie on their stomach on the bed, and position their legs close together, and penetrate from behind. This position will feel great to the non-dominate partner because of the tighter entryway for penetration.

Doggy-Style Stairs – Doing the doggy on the stairs is the perfect set up if you and your spouse wish to perform anal and/or vaginal sex as you take advantage of the incline. It is recommended to lay down a towel or perform this position on carpeted stairs to lean your knees on. The stairs allow your partner to keep themselves upright as you have the power of an upright angle to enter her vagina with.

Hyper-Connected Doggy – For this position, the male or dominant party stands firmly on the floor at the edge of a bed, and the woman or non-dominant gets themselves into the typical doggy-style position. Once the dominant party has entered the un-dominant, they pull their partner up towards them so that they are now kneeling on their knees in front of them. It allows for deep penetration, but also ensures that you can connect with your partner during intercourse.

Chicken-Wing Doggy – This one is funny sounding but rather simplistic. Start in the typical doggy-style position, but lift up her thighs as you thrust in and out of your partner. Ensure that your arm and/or hand is underneath their legs for direct support.

Superhero – If you want to test your strength during intercourse, the superman is a superb way to do such! Let your partner lie upon a table or desk that is sturdy enough for her to support herself. Enter them, and lift their pelvis up slowly so that their feet are off the ground. Let them wrap their feet around your butt if needed. This one is pretty physical, but can be quite the adrenaline rush as you both get close to climax.

Woman on Top Positions

The last two sections allows the man or dominant partner remain in control. Now it is time for the women to take the reigns! These positions offer a nice variety of intimacy as well as female dominance.

Reverse and crouching reverse cowgirl – Dominant party on bottom and subordinate party on top, the cowgirl itself is quite the popular position. The reverse allows the woman to remain in control of the angle of penetration, and the man gets an amazing view of her genitals from behind. The crouching reverse cowgirl is similar, but the woman leans down, for an even better chance of deep penetration. The man can see everything as he watches his penis goes in and out of her.

Woman Lying on Top – There is quite a bit of physical need to accurately perform this position, and it is a great one for those that like anal sex. The woman has the majority of control in this scenario, as she is lying flat on her back as her partner grabs her by the hips. She arches her back and lowers herself up and down, controlling just how deep her partner goes inside her.

Waterfall - This position is not for the couple that is faint of heart, and it may be one of the strangest ones out there. But once you actually master it, one will know why it is worth trying out! As a variation of the cowgirl, the male partner lays on a bed or couch with their head on the edge and their partner on top of them. Once she is mounted on your penis, you will need to slide down off the couch or bed so that your head and shoulders are touching the floor, ensuring that you keep you hips elevated. The woman has total control over speed and penetration deepness. Also, you have two free hands for her or you to do whatever you want with!

Oral Positions

Genital sex is great but not the only option. Whether you are giving it, receiving it or both at the same time, when it comes to cunnilingus, you cannot go wrong! Plus, many females report enjoying it way more than penetration itself.

Lying Down for Him or Her – The least amount of work that either of you have to do sexual wise that still leads to great pleasure lies in the comfort and longevity of this position. Whether it is him lying and her giving a blowjob or licking his ball sac, or her lying down and him pleasuring her clitoris area with his tongue, simple oral stimulation goes a long way, so do not take it lightly!

Standing for Him and Her – Women pleasuring a man's genitals as her stands in front of her kneeling body is possibly one of the most viewed angles during pornography. If it a superb option if a bed or other surface is not available to lie down on. Men can also thrust into the mouths of their partners, with permission of course. And for women, it is a bit trickier for men to ear them out standing up, but it is still a doable option if there is no where suitable to lay her down. Just make sure she spreads her legs a bit for you.

Face Sitting for Him and Her – Having your partner sit on your face and vice versa can be a very attractive way to perform oral sex. It gives both parties and extra sense of either dominance or submissiveness. Have one partner lie on their back and thrust your penis into her mouth, gently. And for her, have her position herself to where her clitoris area is in an easy to reach spot for your entire mouth.

69 – There are a few sexually enticing variations of the classic 69 that can suit and couples' needs.

- **Classic** – Regular 69ing is something that is literally felt from head to toe. Lying on top of one another, each having their heads near the other's crotch areas, it tests the concentration of both partners, for as your give pleasure you are also receiving it.
- **Sideways 69** – Same concept as the classic 69, but you perform it with your partner while lying on your sides. This is a better option for couples who do not feel as comfortable lying on top of each other.

- **Upside down 69** – For those that want to be more adventurous and try something than the average 69ing positions, THIS is the one for you! This variation is not for beginners, and you will need the help of a chin-up bar or something similar that can hold up your body weight. Have one partner get themselves up on the bar, and hang upside down, as the other partner pleasures them orally.

Elevated Cunnilingus – Whether it be on a countertop, in a windowsill or upon a table, you can push your partner onto just about anything that sturdy and take her to town as you pleasure her with your tongue and mouth. Get it on in public! You do not need a bed for this superb position.

Doggy Style Oral – This position is primarily performed on women, as you bend her over a bed or other surface and pleasure her orally from behind. It is also a great way to perform analingus as well.

Standing Positions

There is something to be said not just about variation of the sex positions themselves, but in how we position our bodies to get it on. Instead of the typical bed, it can be super exciting to try some positions that involve you both standing up! It also will assist in your both burning a few more calories than if you were to get it on in bed.

Against the wall – It is extremely hot, especially in the heat of the moment, to push your spouse a little roughly against a wall, pick them up and penetrate them. This is a scene that if often seen in sexy movies, and involves two people who are passionately in love and embracing for usually the firs time. It lets the dominant partner have superb access to their partners neck and breasts for greater sexual pleasure as they are penetrating them.

Standing from behind – If you cannot wait to get it on at home, this position is one that is possible in the midst of a public place, just outside the public eye, of course. This one can also work well for anal sex, too. It is simple, as you are both standing as the dominant partner enters from behind. Having a wall or tree to lean against is recommended, for the submissive partner can take on the deeper thrusts this way.

Woman on table – This position results in great thrusting sex that has a lot of power behind it. Have partner lie upon a table or other flat surface with her butt positioned on the edge of the surface. Enter her, and feel how much power you have this way! Let her put her leg up and resting on your chest or shoulders.

Pile Driver – Out of the hundreds of sex positions out there, this one is among the hardest, but is also super worth it. Both partners must be semi flexible, and neither is likely to go in this position for very long. Have your partner lie on her back, then lift her legs until her torso is off the floor. Straddle her butt once it is above her head, and use a gently up and down motion to enter her vagina.

Sitting and Kneeling Positions

These positions are great for those couples that really want to spice up their love life on a passionate and highly intimate level.

Seated sex – Pull out a comfy chair for this position! Hell, call it for your sex chair if you want! Sit in a sturdy chair with both of your feet planted firmly on the floor. Have your partner straddle you are they face you. Let them lower themselves on top of you, this way she is the one mainly in control and can also tease you as she danced her genitalia on your junk.

Kneeling sex – Even though this position's title sounds like a waste of time, it can be a great one if done correctly. Positioning yourselves in a kneeling position on a yoga mat or other softened surface will make it much more comfortable. It also helps it the two having sex are around the same height. One of you must kneel and place your stretched out knee to the left of your partner as your right knee is holding you up. Your partner does the same. Lower your pelvic bone beneath your partner's and graciously put your penis inside her.

The Bridge – This position gives great views of the dominant's partner. The dominant person kneels, while the submissive person creates an arch, or bridge, with their arms and legs and kneels in front of dominate as they penetrate them. The view of their breasts and body as they have the chance to grab their hips and thrust against them is quite epic and a turn on all the same.

Unusual Positions

These diverse sexual positions are definitely for the faint of heart. These are meant for those couples that really want to get down and dirty and try new things that are outside their comfort zones.

Wheelbarrow – It is time to get physical with this sex position! It is ALL about how much upper body strength you possess as well as how much your back and legs can take. Have your partner get on all fours, and then proceed to lift their pelvis up high enough for the other partner to insert their penis inside. The submissive person acts as the 'wheelbarrow.'

Surfboard – This position involves a bathtub that is big enough to fit both you and your partner. Fill the tub about halfway with water, but do not fill it much more than that. The dominant partner sits within the bathtub and relaxes with his legs extended out. The submissive person sits on top of the other and is the one that does most of the work, kind of like in surfing. The water surrounding your bodies will feel great! But keep in mind that water will wash away any lubrication that may have been present when you got in the tub.

Sit and Spin – Take advantage of the vibrations that your washer or dryer puts out by having your partner sit on top of you as you thrust. It is an added sensation that is unlike anything else!

There are of course MANY other sexual positions to try out there, but this a good list to get you started in your exciting sexual ventures!

Mastering the G-Spot

Despite popular belief among a broad range of men, a woman's G-spot is not a myth; it is a realistic part of her sexuality. The problem is the fact that many do not know what they are looking for when it comes to successfully locating their spouse's g-spot, let alone how to use it to their advantage once they DO find it. This sacred spot within the vagina is not like the clitoris, for there are some women that actually do not find much pleasure when it is located and fondled with. Thankfully, for the majority of women, when people find this spot and know how to coddle it to perfection, it assists in the development of mind blowing orgasms.

If you are one that struggles in finding a women's G-spot, you are not alone. It is by far one of life's mysteries, and even sex-perts argue over the existence of the g-spot, and if it even is present in ALL women. They do know one thing: When sexed right, the g-spot is the trigger point to make women go absolutely insane.

So, what IS the G-spot exactly? It is a sensitive area that is located just inside the front wall of the vagina. And when it is played with and/or stimulated correctly, it can help bring a female to orgasm faster than it they just performed penetrative intercourse. It is kind of like a lock box, you must figure out the combination to get it to open up to the results you want. The orgasms that result from g-spot stimulation are different than that of clitoral stimulated orgasms. G-spot pleasure is felt from deep within the vagina, which is why women who experience it love it so much!

How to Find a Women's G-Spot

First, PLEASE wash your hands. No one wants a pair of grimy hands all up in their personal business. Also ensure that your fingernails are trimmed and filed down, because another terrible thing is getting cut up by nasty, sharp nails. You are exploring very sensitive places here, please take these steps to heart and use them wisely. Fingers are by far the best way to locate a g-spot, due to the fact that they fit well inside and have the ability to move in different directions.

There is no way your lady's vagina is just going to let you RIGHT into its fortress. You are going to have to conduct some good foreplay before you even dare enter, for you will need the proper natural lubrication to pleasure your lady as your locate her lockbox and figure out the code. Foreplay before trying to find her secret treasure also allow the g-spot to swell in size as she becomes aroused, making it a piece of cake to find later!

The G-spot is usually located about 2 inches inside the vagina, on the top of the vaginal wall. It is best for you to finger your partner with her lying comfortably on her back, and insert a finger with your palm facing upwards. When you have gently entered her, start to make a "come here" motion with your finger, and you should feel a textured area in the shape of a bean around the zone explained above. If you find that, you are on the fast track to help your partner ride the pleasure train. You may want to have your lady lift up her knees to her chest so that your fingers and hand has more room to access her g-spot as well.

Body language is the core lingo to pay attention to during any type of sexual play or intercourse. It is the tall tale sign if she likes what you are doing to her. Listen to her noises and moans and watch her facial expressions and how her body tenses up. You will know whether or not she is enjoying herself or wants you to get away from her. Stimulating the g-spot has the same concepts of when you penetrate her. You do not roughly thrust your junk inside her, you do so smoothly, gently and slowly, taking time to figure out a good rhythm that works great for both of you. The same goes for locating and stimulating her g-spot.

Ensure that she likes what you are doing to her. If she is not providing enough feedback to get an accurate reading of her body language, talk to her and ask her how she feels, and make changes according to her desires and wants. Do not take lack of feedback as an invitation to increase pressure or pace. There is a chance that she does not know much about her own g-spot, or may just not like the sensation of it being stimulated like other women do. That does not mean you should give up on mastering her g-spot. Hell, it may take a few attempts before the g-spot gives way to the pleasure you are trying to provide it! And your lady may not even know the amount of pleasure she could receive from your future attempts.

Once you do work your way up to gaining her g-spot's trust and your partner likes your technique, a tip is to use your free hand while your other is stimulating the g-spot to press gently down on the area of her belly just about her pubic area. This gently pressure can help stimulate the g-spot even further. Once you get her riled up to a certain point with your fingers, it is time top try sexual positions such as the class doggy style, that directly make contact with her g-spot.

How to Last Longer in the Sack

It is kind of hard to believe that with all the unique sexual positions, props and other sexual gadgets, that the average time that actual intercourse lasts is 5 to 7 minutes, with another huge portion only lasting 2 minutes! What?! With those statistics, it is safe to say that both men and women would like their sex to last much longer, with the ideal length for many being 10 – to 25 minutes. This chapter is full of knowledgeable ways to spend more time being sexually playful in the sack, rather than picking up the embarrassing pieces and mere disappointment afterwards.

Ways to Broaden Your Man's Stamina

Numbing agents – This one may take a bit of skill to perform correctly, and should be done with care, for it can get messy at the drop of a hat. Numbing sprays that come in contact directly with a man's penis are the easiest routes to take. And once put inside the woman, the female party will not feel the numbing agent running off on her.

Perpendicular positions – This is a great way to avoid those really sensitive, erogenous zones of the penis. Instead of letting him penetrate you, do the work of gliding back and forth along the shaft of the penis. Face each other or spoon while laying on your sides. This will assist him not immediately rush to orgasm.

Kegels?! – Yes, men can do kegels too! Kegels along with Pilates or yoga all help strengthen his pelvic floor muscles, which will then assist him in controlling the spasms that come along with orgasming.

Squeeze base of penis – Utilizing a cock ring or just your hand, use a firm grip and grasp the base of his dong. It will literally prevent him from ejaculating.

Edging – When your man informs you that he is about to come, make him stop and then wait patiently for about a minute or two before sticking his penis back inside you. Edging allow his body to get used to delaying the inevitable act of ejaculation. And while he is waiting, that gives him plenty of opportunity to please you!

Make it awkward – Especially if you have been with your partner for some time, you may have developed a slight routine, which allows his body to literally anticipate coming, and makes him do so a lot sooner than you both would like. Trying out new positions, routines and sensations will distract him, allowing him to last longer without really even realizing it. The more awkward the new things you try, the better.

Masturbate before intercourse – have your man masturbate and ejaculate about one to two hours before you anticipate having sex. This way, when arousal is built up later, your guys' satisfaction has already been somewhat fulfilled so he can learn to better pace himself and get in rhythm with you, his partner. Regular masturbation is indeed healthy and allows men to perform longer in bed as well.

'Cool down' methods – There are a couple proven techniques that you can learn and teach yourself to prevent the possibility of pre-ejaculation and orgasming too quickly. Some of these techniques, however, will have to be practiced before you can use them during the course of sex. Otherwise they will not work to their highest potential.

- **TBP Method** – TBP refers to tongue, back and push. Take your tongue and run the tip of it in a circle motion on the top of your mouth. You can do this with your mouth closed so that your partner doesn't have to know you are utilizing this method. As you are moving your tongue, run yours hands along your partner's back in elongated strokes. Stroke from her shoulders to her lower back. Really take the time to feel the texture of their skin during this process. The final step is to utilize your PC muscle, pushing it out as much as you can comfortably. Push and release the tension that you are feeling. Hold for a few seconds and then release. Then relax for another few seconds. Do the last step a few times until you feel the tension that has built up settle back out.

- **Snooze button method** – This method is one that should be used as a LAST resort, because it involves the manual prevention of ejaculation. The thing that men do not realize is that there is a keen difference between ejaculation and the actual action of having an orgasm. This method is used to just prevent the action of ejaculating, not stopping an orgasm itself. In this method, you will need to find the midway point between your anus and your balls. When you feel yourself starting to reach the climax stage, firmly hold this place down. Some contracting will occur, but make sure to hold this place down firmly until they cease.

Communication – Taking the time to speak up and talk to your partner can go a long ways in gaining confidence and figuring out a plan to last a little longer during sex. Men are usually pretty reluctant to talk to their partners about their sexual shortcomings. Women will think that you do not care about their sexual needs if you never can talk about your issues.

Switch focus – You need to stop putting so much emphasis on your performance and think more about the moments you are taking part in sexually instead. If you start to be more concerned about how long you can last in bed, then that is all your mind will think about, further inhibiting your longevity during intercourse.

How to Please Your Man in Bed

Despite the fact that males manage to get turned on faster and more efficiently time wise than females, it takes more than just a simple touch or rub down to really get your man satisfied. Learning how to sexually fulfill your partner is an art all on its own, and it is a practice you need to hone sooner rather than later if you want your sexual buddy to stick around. Within this chapter you will get brushed up on some sex basics, as well as learn some new-fangled approaches that men have kept secrets from women that lead to the path of total pleasure for them. These tips are straightforward, and you can see results from acting upon them in a matter of mere days!

Foreplay – We have already discussed this tip, in fact, it filled up an entire first chapter! Arousing your partner in creative, sexual ways will keep them wanting to be dominant for a longer period of time. Use these further foreplay tips:

- **Do not underestimate background music** – Having soothing, romantic or risqué tunes will be a good fire to get the mood going. You may be surprised how it can mentally and physically set the mood for you both.
- **Put your tongue to work** – you can awake your partners senses if you kiss and taunt him with your tongue all over his body
- **Fondle gently** – He will love that he is deemed untouchable by you! I promise you

Relax – Sex is supposed to be a FUN venture. You must be creative when it comes to delivering successful activities in the sack to your man, to constantly keep him intrigued. Here are some tips to help make bedroom games more fun:

- **Experiment with positions** – It is okay to be a little nervous at first when trying out new sexual positions, but remember to go with the flow and have fun with it! Your man will be glad you want to try out cool new things with him, and that in itself will boost his confidence.

- **Healthy competition** – A little bit of competition between you and your hubby can go a long ways when it comes to the world of sex. Challenge one another into seeing who can get who to orgasm quicker.

Hone your oral skills – Having the capability to satisfy your man with just your mouth is a good quality to have! When done successfully, he will have amazing orgasms that he will only want to thank you for later. Here are some orally given tips to keep in mind when going down on your guy:

- Concentrate on giving him pleasure by stimulating the more sensitive areas of his penis, mainly the tip. You will also need to pay attention to the entirety of the penis as a whole. The entire thing is filled with truckloads of nerve endings that are just anticipating your tongue rolling over them.
- Ensure to use tons of saliva while sucking on his organ. This will assist in stimulating him in the right way for him to feel more pleasured.

Stimulate his mind – It has been mentioned a few times within this book already that for an intensely great sexual experience you must be in the mood physically and mentally. And what better way to get your guy in the mood than turning on your sexy tone of voice and talking dirty to him? This is a sure fire way to get him aroused rather quick like. Here are some great ideas in what to say in that naughty tone of voice that is within all of us women:
- "I love the way you taste"
- "I can not wait for you to be inside me."
- "Shall we go ahead with this?"

Positivity – Instilling a positive state of mind and attitude is not just something that we should have in our daily lives, it is something that should also be taken with us to the bedroom in the heat of the moment. Be enthusiastic, no matter what your goal is for that point in time. Ensure that you are clearly stating that you are wanting and cannot wait to have sexual intercourse with him. He will play off of this attitude ten fold, which is better for you ladies in the long run! Here are some tips in making sure he knows you are ready to pounce:

- Ensure that you are giving off the right types of body language. Sensually moving in bed or while you get in bed is a great way to do this.
- Jump into the sack earlier than he does. This way he knows you are turned on and wanting them to make that first move.

Turn fantasies into reality – Besides bringing in a classy smile and a good attitude to bed, every once in a while you will need to explore the realm of other possibilities sex wise, such as making his fantasies that I am sure he plays over and over in his mind a reality for him and you! It will be easy to satisfy his fantasy if you talk to him about it, and get a true sense what his fantasy driven desires actually include. Here are some tips to get to know his fantasies and what he wants out of them:

- Ask about his fantasies when the time is right. Do not judge what he tells you either! This will kill that buzz for him automatically.
- Once you have a good idea, you can gradually try out new things that relate to that fantasy. He will also gradually start to share more and more with you as well after you have already asked about it once.

How to Please your Woman in Bed

And now it is time to retract the statement that the process of truly satisfying a person in bed is in art. Well, it is, but it is for men. To satisfy women, it takes quality time to delve into a deeper understanding of who they are as people and what their needs and desires are. If you put a women's sexual needs and desires ahead of yours, you are on the right track to making her fall in love with you sexually, for this will keep both of your guys' sex lives alive for a long time coming.

Again, undoubtedly the most powerful sex organ in our bodies does not reside in our undies, it is locked away in our craniums! A woman's brain plays an especially vital role in getting her into the mood to get down and dirty. If your brain is informing you that you are having phenomenal sex, then the other parts of your body will follow suit right behind it, leading to amazing bouts of pleasure. This is how you will forever and successfully satisfy any woman in bed, unlocking the mental secrets that will make her moldable under your sexual ruling.

The following are great tips to lead to your ladies' ultimate satisfaction while playing with one another in the sheets.

Create the perfect orgasm – No, this is not impossible to accomplish, but it does take a certain skill set to be successful at it. Orgasms occur during the grand climax of lovemaking, and if you end up retrieving the big O before she manages to do so, she will more than likely never reach climax and live without her big finish. Learning to control your erection goes hand in hand (no pun intended) in making sure your lady reaches the edge of satisfaction.

Suck, nibble, bite and lick – Kissing is a super intimate and romantic turn on, but there is no need to stop using your mouth and all the capabilities it has to offer her body at her lips, no no! Let her feel the passion that is flowing through you for her all throughout her body as your tongue your way down it. Love bites in erogenous regions are a sure fire way to turn her on heavily to you.

Sex refreshers – Sex can tend to become a repetitive and seem like more of a chore after awhile. That is why it is beyond crucial to mix things up and add different kinds of foreplay, as well as role playing in with sex. Dirty talking and playing sexily fun games that turn you both on are great ways to achieve a change of pace in the bedroom.

Play with her body – When your penis is inside of her, do not forget that the rest of her body need not go untouched! Play with parts of her body as you thrust in and out of her. Stroke, grab and massage her in all the areas she likes. It will continuously turn your girl on than your and your penis have a one track mind mission and goal set.

Compliment her – Women are complimentary beings who love feeling appreciated, as well as the sound of a well thought out compliment. It will get them to experiment with you sooner on new things you wish to try as well. Do not hold your thoughts back. Make sure to inform her of how well she looks in her new lingerie, or how great her breasts feel. It will give her a mighty confidence boost, making her a better playmate sex wise.

Do not be afraid to experiment – If you and your lady are all about getting in on missionary style all the time, it is bound to become awfully boring. Experiment with new positions, fun toys and dirty conversations. It is best to attempt to try new things as often as possible, so your sex life does not become stale. Because trust me, there is NO fun in that.

Be selfless – Ensure that you are constantly trying to put your lady's needs ahead of your own. It is of good practice to have a deepened understanding of her bedside preferences. Ensure that she is always feeling comfortable in her skin around you, otherwise she will not enjoy you near as much as if she is totally comfortable with everything you do and want to achieve sexually.

Whisper sweet nothings – Women have vividly active imaginations and rely on them more than visual representations, unlike men. Arouse her by utilizing the right words. Whisper dirty thoughts into her ear, and talk about your guys' shared fantasies. Excite her brain with beyond seductive vocabulary.

Keep it clean – ensure that you are taking care of yourself to look good for your woman. Hygiene plays an important role in how women feel about you, especially since you want to get inside them as soon as you can. A better looking partner is more of a turn on than one who doesn't take the time and energy to care for themselves.

Do not drift to sleep – Heading into lala dream land right after you do the deed is not attractive whatsoever. Take the time after sex to talk about what just happened, or to catch up on you and your partner's day. I guess in secure relationships, falling asleep is a decent sign, because that means you are both gracious enough to enjoy each other and relax after such a rush of sensations, rather than worrying about awkwardness and how they felt about the sex you gave them.

Do not forget the erogenous regions – There are quite a few highly sensitive areas among the body of a typical woman. Ensure that you take time to explore her body in its entirety. Each woman has a set of different sweet spots than the next that you can really take advantage of.

Go on! Go downtown! – If anything else fails in arousing your lady, going down on her will usually always do the trick. If you are having issues getting her warmed up and ready for intercourse with you, take a sweet allotted amount of time to tongue your way around her vagina, especially her clitoris. This will help build up a decent amount of momentum to get you two started.

Let's Talk Oral

It is important for both men and women to realize, accept and conquer the major differences that both sexes have when it comes to giving and receiving oral sex. For men, oral sex is quite simple, and can be one of the more relaxing states of intercourse as a whole. Most men are the same as to what they desire when receiving oral from women. Women, however, are a wee bit more complicated, however. Cunnilingus for her is like figuring out the combination to all of her sexual goodness the difficult way, for every single woman is distinctly particular about what they desire and want from their man while they are all up in their downtown business. This chapter will unlock some of the secrets of what both sexes ACTUALLY crave when it comes to the subject of oral sex. Some of these may just surprise you!

Oral Tips to try on Men

The goal of giving oral is to provide the best pleasure filled experience to them as you possibly can. The funny thing? There are many people who do not bother to communicate about what they like and would rather have you not do when it comes to their most sensitive areas of their body. Here are some amazing tips that will hopefully blow your man's mind if done the right way! But honestly, you kind of HAVE to try to go wrong with these. Easy peasy!

Lights out – For some reason, when women are in the process of sucking off their partner, the lights burning before them make them uncomfortable. Just shut the lights out! It will give your guy a whole new sense of pleasure, as you are invisible to him.

Gag-free tip – Many women dislike giving oral to men because of the fear of gagging and essentially puking on them. Gross. And a mood killer. Take the tip of your tongue and place it along the roof of your mouth, and let his privates actually hit the underside of your tongue. Gag-free!

Give the other boys attention – Men often complain that their women totally ignore their balls during the course of oral and sex in general. While you take one hand to pleasure the shaft of his penis, use you mouth to pleasure one of his testicles at a time as you lightly suck it in and out of your mouth.

Use some pressure – There is one area that women and even some men do not realize has super sensitive potential. The hole at the tip of the penis, called the meatus, is hyper sensitive. If you take the tip of your tongue and add some pressure to that spot as you lick it, it will drive your guy nuts.

Lube him up – If you plan to orally pleasure him for awhile, get some good tasting lube! If will make it much more fun for both of you, without the nasty task of constantly spitting on him to keep his penis wet.

Missing this spot – Take your tongue and trail down the shaft of his penis, the area that is between his balls and the base of the penis. Purse your lips and lightly suck on this patch of skin. It is filled with many nerve endings, so giving it any kind of attention will get him going.

F-Spot – Isn't it amazing just how many erogenous spots are on a man's penis?! Here is another! The bump right underneath where the shaft meets the tip, called the frenulum, or the F-spot, likes attention too! Take the tip of a finger on it and place it there, then put both his shaft and your finger in your mouth and move up and down as you continuously add pressure to the F-spot. He will love you.

Visual appeal – Men are already naturally visual creatures, so place a mirror next to you when you are getting down and dirty so he can check you out as you pleasure him.

Oral Tips to try on Women

Women are unique masterpieces, built slightly complicated in many aspects besides sexually, one of the things that makes women interesting and intriguing to men. Men find it to be their mission to unlock the secrets of the way women function, especially in bed. Many men hard core struggle giving proper oral to their ladies, so this section will be mighty helpful! If you are a woman that purchased this book, you may want to "accidentally" leave this open somewhere in the house where he will come across it.

Take it slow – Do not, by any means, go straight to her vagina and start going to town on her. BAD. Take your time, making pit stops on your way down her body. Take plenty of time pleasuring her other erogenous zones before parking the care downtown. Women LOVE a buildup of tension.

Self –Consciousness – Women are super, crazily self-conscious about the way their vaginas taste and smell. Ensure that you use your words and proper body language when going down on her. Tell her she is beautiful, and they you cannot wait to eat her gorgeous vagina out.

Gentle – use every part of your mouth, be creative by all means! But do NOT use your teeth, in any circumstance. It will do nothing but hurt her.

Listen – If you hear nothing coming from her, such as sexually moaning or sounds, you are doing something wrong. Soften your touch a bit, go to a different area and listen again. If you hear her moaning, you found a good spot and should stick to it.

Helping hands – Your tongue feels amazing, but do not be afraid to add in some finger action too! Just remember to not act as if your hand is a jackhammer. Be gentle, and ensure that you insert or use fingers when she is well lubricated.

Everyone is different – Do not do all the things that your ex-girlfriend told you to do with your new girl. Every woman is vastly different, you will need to take time to explore her and find what she likes. Sorry, no short cuts here!

Clitoral Action – For God's sake, if you are not already knowledgeable, figure out where her darn clitoris is! It is the sanctuary of pleasure for her. It is the small bump at the top of the vagina, and may be hiding behind her clitoral hood. But do not spend all your time at the clit, browse along her entire vagina. The entirety of it is filled with pleasurable nerve endings.

Suck away – do not be afraid to suck gently down there in various places. She will enjoy the different motions you are making with your mouth.

Utilize different speeds – Do not just go slow or fast the entire time, because you will continuously fail at getting her off orally. Speed it up, slow it down, and use variety! She will enjoy it, I promise.

There are hundreds of other cool and unique tips on giving great oral stimulation to both men and women. Change up your routine on your partner and start using some of these TONIGHT. You would be surprised at how much better it will be for both of you!

Sexual Massages

If you want a way to get really intimate with your partner and get them in the mood, sexual massages are great ways to do so. Massages are tried and true ways to continuously keep things exciting in the bedroom setting. So it is important to know a few techniques to keep within your sleeve to use, for if you do not know what you are doing, it definitely takes the allure out of it.

Massages are all about getting each of you relaxed, taking minds off of the course of your day and getting both of you in the zone to truly take in and absorb one another. It can be a big part of foreplay, and if done right, might end up as the favorite part of play before intercourse!

Set the Mood – The right kind of atmosphere is crucial to setting the mood the right way! Ambience is everything, and it will determine just how long your partner will feel relaxed as your massage them.

- **Play music** – Find relaxing music, or even play your favorites, just ensure that it is kept at a low volume.
- **Nice smell** – Grab some scented candles and light them before they come in, so that the room smells wonderfully.
- **Temperature** – You do not want a room that is too hot or too cold, make sure it is comfortable naked.
- **Get a towel** – Ensure that you are not going to get the bed all messy where you will be having intercourse later. Conduct massage on towel.
- **Dim lights** – Dimmer switches come in handy for this, but if you are not so lucky, get a couple table lamps that have dimmer lighting qualities.

Grab some essential oils – Quality oils are a crucial piece of sensual massages, and it is just as important to choose the right ones. They smell wonderful and adequately lubricate the skin.

- **Sandalwood oil** – Assists in increasing libido
- **Rose oil** – Smells great and is known for creating a sense of romance

- **Grapeseed oil** – The best one for many, doesn't irritate skin as you massage

Massage Techniques – While honing your massage techniques, ALWAYS ensure that you have plenty of oil upon yours hands. Use circular movements that eventually turn into long glides and then back to circular movements that are short in length. Continue to use variations of both of these throughout massage. If you feel knots within their body, make sure to take extra time on these areas, for they are physically and obviously tense. You want them to be less stiff and soft.

- **Back** – Focus on the legs, butt, lower and upper back for 15 minutes. Then start at the shoulders and arms and move down them. Spend around 2 or 3 minutes on these areas.

- **Front** – Ask them nicely to turn over and keep their eyes closed, to ensure relaxation. Massage their breasts, arms, stomach and legs. You can massage their feet too, but make sure they actually like this. For some it might be too ticklish to actually relax them. Spend 2 or 3 minutes on each of these areas of their bodies.

- **Lower areas** – With the rest of the body fully relaxed and all massaged up, you can now massage genital areas and the regions surrounding their privates, gently and slowly. When you hear a moan or two, you can insert fingers or really start to rub more vigorously, ensuring that you have plenty of oil for lubrication. Even though, by now, there is probably plenty of natural lubrication. This would be the time to make a move for the F-spot on him and the G-spot on her.

Keep in Mind...

- If you want to beef up massages, run a tub full of hot water that you can both sit in afterwards. After washing off all that oil sexual wise, you can hit the bedroom.
- 100% organic based oils are best. They last longer and are thick in consistency, making them unharmful to the skin.
- Test different kinds of pressure and ask them what they like throughout the massage. Ensure that you take things very slow.
- Whisper in their ear occasionally and ask them how they like it. That will turn them on fast.
- Ensure that before you start, that your hands are warm. No one likes to be touched with cold hands. Use oil and rub your hands together for a fw minutes before starting the massaging process.
- When you are massaging, have your partner lie down and sit on or near their butt. This is a turn on for both parties.

Conclusion

Thank for making it through to the end of this sexually intriguing and informative novel. I hope it was able to shed some light on improved ways to enhance your sexual game in the bedroom, as well as successfully pleasing your partner to make them beg for more! The tools, tricks and techniques that your noggin just absorbed will ensure that you will be a sexual challenge to reckon with. I hope that you are now able to achieve your goals of being the passionate erotic person you have always wanted your significant other to have!

The next step is to obviously get busy and try some of these unique and brand new positions and techniques! You may want to inform your partner, or if you choose not to, be prepared at the surprised faces and intimate reactions you are bound to get by making these moves on them in the sack! The only thing I CAN ensure you of is you and your spouse are about to become much closer, and possibly little sexual bunny rabbits! For the knowledge you just soaked up will make you and your companion crave sex more than ever.

With the conclusion of this book, all I have left to say is a big GOOD LUCK in your future sexual endeavors. Congratulations on finally taking the steps by reading this book to take back your sex life. You are your partner are only bound to enjoy every little bit of it!

Finally, if you found this book useful in anyway, a review on Amazon is always appreciated!

Description

Are you tired of being "just average" when it comes to having sex? Have the once amazing carnal techniques that you once had up your sleeve just not doing the trick in satisfying your or your partner anymore? Are you just ready for something excitingly new when it comes to pleasuring and being pleasured? Well, you are in LUCK! The book you have stumbled upon today holds pages upon pages of new-fangled skills that will give you the knowledge to embrace your inner sexual fiend!

Enhancing yourself to be better when it comes to animal-like intimacy comes easy for some and hard for others. The chapters of this book will discuss proven tips, techniques and strategies on the best ways to stimulate your partner for more intense sexual pleasure. This book includes:

- Techniques for phenomenal foreplay
- Approaches to various sexual positions to try out in other places other than the bedroom to spice things up!
- Mastering the location of her G-Spot and how to thrillingly satisfy her with it
- Ways to last longer during intercourse
- How to please your man in bed
- How to please your woman in bed
- How to give amazing oral sex!
- How to perform arousing sexual massages
- And much more!

Even those that are sexually advanced with their partners will benefit from the tips and knowledge that this book has to offer! If you are an individual who is a bit shy to really get down and dirty, this book is written to provide you with the absolute confidence to really get out of your comfort zone and try new things. When it comes to satisfying each other in bed, now a days we lack the commitment to the time we really should be spending literally tasting our spouses or party go-er friends! What is the point of having sex if it does not excite you in some way or another? The last thing you want is for you and your partner's sex life to become boring and stale.

And if the act of sex is starting to seem more like a chore than a fun, physically bonding activity, it is beyond time to spice things up and try new techniques! So, what the heck are ya waiting for?! Purchase this book and get to reading! I promise you that it will be one of the best things you did, and possibly one of the best books your eyes have feasted their eyes upon!

www.ingramcontent.com/pod-product-compliance
Lightning Source LLC
Chambersburg PA
CBHW071306280526
45788CB00004B/1842